HAMMOND PUBLIC LIBRARY

3 1161 00066 5029

WITHDRAWN

'80 0 5 2 9 6   y615.781

D1216967

DATE DUE			
JUL 28 '80			

Shapiro, Irwin
  Gift of magic sleep.

MAIN CHILDREN'S ROOM
Hammond Public Library
Hammond, Ind.

THE GIFT OF MAGIC SLEEP

THE GIFT OF MAGIC SLEEP

Early Experiments in Anesthesia

Irwin Shapiro · illustrated by Pat Rotondo

Coward, McCann & Geoghegan, Inc.
New York

Hammond Public Library
Hammond, Ind.

—'80 05296

5.99

Anesthesia is the greatest gift ever made to suffering humanity.
—Sir William Osler

Text copyright © 1979 by Irwin Shapiro

Illustrations copyright © 1979 by Pat Rotondo

All rights reserved. This book, or parts thereof, may not be reproduced in any form without permission in writing from the publishers. Published simultaneously in Canada by Longman Canada Limited, Toronto.

LIBRARY OF CONGRESS CATALOGING IN PUBLICATION DATA

Shapiro, Irwin. The gift of magic sleep.
Bibliography: p.

SUMMARY: Traces the discovery of anesthesia in the mid–19th century discussing the contributions of the four men most directly responsible, Crawford W. Long, Horace Wells, William T. G. Morton, and Charles T. Jackson.

1. Anesthesia—History—Juvenile literature.
[1. Anesthesia—History] I. Rotondo, Pat. II. Title.
RD79.S53   617'.96   78–24224   ISBN 0–698–30694–5 lib. bdg.

615.781

PRINTED IN THE UNITED STATES OF AMERICA

main

CONTENTS

Y615.781

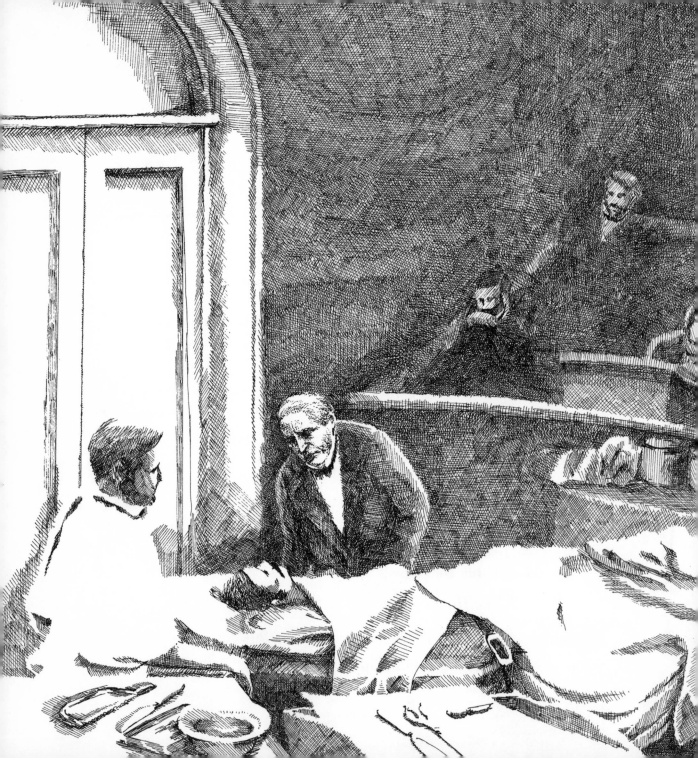

1 · The Knife That Heals

He was a grown man, but his face twisted as though he were a baby about to cry. He was a young man, but his hands trembled as though he were a hundred years old.

Raising his head, he looked around the operating room. It was really an operating theater. Above was a high, domed ceiling; at one end was a steep bank of seats filled with medical students. They were listening to the frock-coated surgeon who stood before them.

He turned slightly and caught sight of the surgeon's instruments. Laid out on a small table, glittering in the light, were knives and saws. He knew they were meant for him, and suddenly he wanted to run.

He wanted to leap up, to rush out—out of this room, out of this hospital, into the street. He wanted to run and run until he was so far away no one could find him.

He could not move. He was flat on his back, strapped tightly to the operating table. Even if he could burst through the straps, the surgeon's assistants would hold him down. And if he could, somehow, throw them off, he still could not run. His right leg, injured in an accident, was swollen with gangrene, and useless. And yet he had to escape, to get away from those knives and saws.

"Doctor," he said to the surgeon, "no. No operation. Let me out of here."

The surgeon touched him gently on the shoulder.

"Steady, now," he said. "I know it's a hard thing to lose a leg, but it will save your life."

"Yes . . . but . . . the pain. . . ."

"I'll be as quick as I can," the surgeon said.

He nodded to an assistant, who lifted up the leg. He applied a tourniquet above the knee, then reached for a knife. The next moment the knife bit into the flesh, and the young man let out a terrible scream.

"No, no!" he cried. "Stop! Please!"

Again and again, as the surgeon worked over him, he screamed and yelled and groaned. He strained against the straps, and three assistants gripped him and held him down.

"Oh, God!" he shouted. "Have mercy! Let me die!"

Blood gushed under the knife, staining the surgeon's hands. A student in the front row gagged and ran from the room. With the screams came the rasp of a saw, the crunch of bone, and the thump of the leg dropping into the tub under the table.

It was over at last. Where the leg had been there was now only a bloody stump. The wound was dressed and the young man, moaning, was wheeled back to his bed.

As the students gathered up their notes and filed out, the surgeon sighed. Yes, the operation was over—and still those terrible screams

8

seemed to hang in the air. Washing the blood from his hands, he shook his head. He had done his best. There was no other way to operate. The knife that heals, he told himself, must first give pain.

The surgeon was Dr. John Collins Warren; the hospital, Massachusetts General in Boston. Dr. Warren was a famous surgeon. He was dean of Harvard Medical School and one of the founders of the hospital. But he might have been any surgeon in any hospital in the world, for the year was 1844. Anesthetics—drugs that relieve pain—were unknown. The patient was fully conscious during every second of the operation.

No wonder, Dr. Warren thought, that many people choose to die rather than suffer such pain. And even if an operation were successful, the patient might die from shock. More than one man, faced with an amputation, said, "I'd sooner die whole." No wonder, too, that doctors were not eager to operate. In the last five years, only 184 operations had been performed at Massachusetts General, an average of about three a month.

Slowly Dr. Warren walked to his office, closed the door, and sat down. He was tired, tired; his arms felt heavy and lifeless. To give as little pain as possible, he had tried to work fast. All surgeons worked fast. The best surgeon, they said, was the fastest surgeon. And the operations had to be simple, such as the removal of tumors and the amputation of arms and legs. No surgeon dared to go deeply into the patient's body. It was too painful, too dangerous.

Not that operations were anything new. Men had been practicing surgery for centuries—and for centuries they had been searching for ways to relieve pain. They had tried drugs made from various plants.

They had tried alcohol, in the form of wine and whiskey. They had tried pressure on a nerve. They had tried a method of hypnotism called mesmerism. None of these was sure enough or safe enough.

They were still trying. Why, hardly a week passed without someone coming to Dr. Warren with some great new discovery, some magic way of putting patients to sleep.

"Magic," he muttered. "Humbugs, that's what they are. If only there really was a magic sleep. . . ."

Through the open window came the clop-clop of horses' hooves, the creak of carriage wheels, the shouts of children playing. And over them all he seemed to hear again the screams and yells and groans of the operating room.

He shook his head. Surgery could heal, but the operating room was a place of torture. Must there always be such suffering? Was there no way in the world to relieve such pain?

2 · Sweet Vitriol and Laughing Gas

Ever since the beginning of surgery, thousands of doctors, like Dr. Warren, had wished there were a magic sleep. And countless patients, facing the horror of an operation, had had the same wish. And yet, the drugs that could produce such a sleep—ether and nitrous oxide—had been known for many years. They had been discovered and forgotten, rediscovered and again forgotten, time after time after time.

Ether, a compound of sulphuric acid and alcohol, had been discovered by an alchemist as early as the thirteenth century. Because it resembled other compounds called vitriol, and had a rather sweet smell, it was called sweet vitriol.

No one knew what use it had, and for several hundred years it was forgotten. Then a physician named Paracelsus rediscovered sweet vitriol. He experimented with it on chickens, noting that they "fall asleep for a long time, awaking undamaged." He recommended that it be used for "painful illnesses."

Although sweet vitriol was included in a list of all known medicines published in Germany in 1542, no one seemed interested. Not until the eighteenth century was it mentioned by such scientists as Sir Isaac Newton and Robert Boyle. In 1792 a German chemist became interested in sweet vitriol and renamed it ether.

Meanwhile, in 1772, the English chemist Joseph Priestley had discovered nitrous oxide. He also discovered oxygen and other gases. He experimented on mice with pure oxygen, believing it might be used to treat diseases of the lung. Inhaling it himself, he found that it gave him "a remarkable sense of freedom and lightness in the chest."

Before Priestley, little had been known about gases. His discoveries, and his book, *Experiments and Observations Concerning the Different Kinds of Air*, gave doctors an idea.

Up to this time, they had had only one way of giving patients medicines—by mouth. Priestley showed them a new way—by inhalation. They began using gases to treat diseases, mostly diseases of the lung, such as asthma. They tried oxygen, hydrogen, and nitrogen. Some even tried ether. The one gas they refused to try was nitrous oxide. They did experiment with it on animals, with bad results. Nitrous oxide was a poison, they decided, and could cause death.

It was a seventeen-year-old boy who proved them wrong. He was Humphrey Davy, a doctor's apprentice in England. One day he heard several doctors discussing the dangers of nitrous oxide, and he made up his mind to find out more about it.

Alone, at night, he made some nitrous oxide. Was it really as dangerous as they said? Could it really kill? Well, he would soon know.

He took a breath of the gas—and he did not die. He took another breath, and another and another—and still he did not die. Instead, he seemed to be floating, floating in the air like a feather. He felt

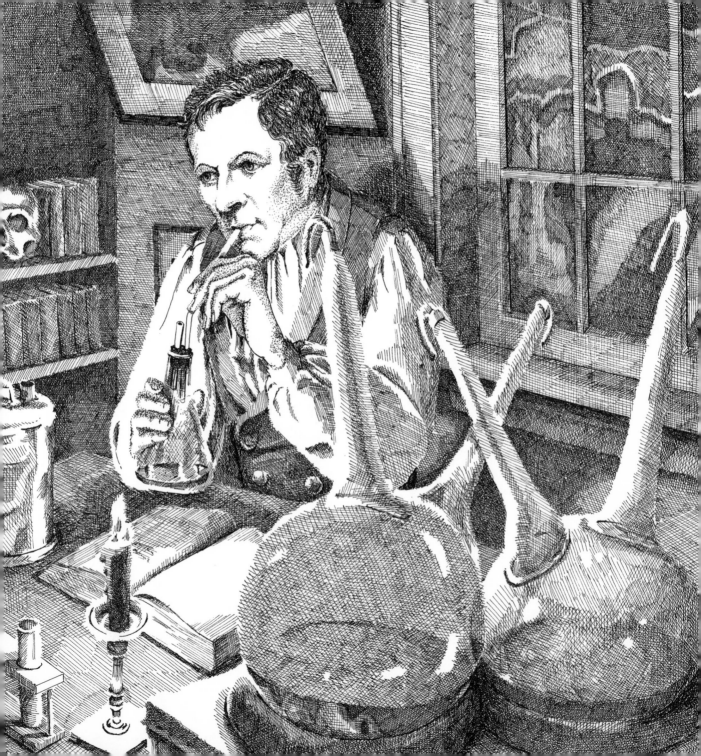

wonderfully cheerful, and burst out laughing. He could not help himself. He had to laugh, and he could not stop laughing until the effect of the gas wore off.

Night after night he inhaled the gas, each time with the same result. He decided that it was dangerous only if taken in too large a dose.

And one night he discovered something else. He happened to be cutting a wisdom tooth; his gums were hot and swollen, and he was in great pain. He inhaled the gas, and the pain was dulled. So—nitrous oxide could relieve pain.

The following year Davy took a position at Dr. Thomas Beddoes's Pneumatic Institute. There patients with lung diseases were treated by the inhalation of various gases. Davy went on experimenting with nitrous oxide, which was soon called "laughing gas."

Davy's work at the Institute made him widely known. When he was twenty-two he became a lecturer on chemistry at the Royal Institution, which had been formed for the study of science. Crowds flocked to his lectures, and many noted people tried inhaling his laughing gas. For a few minutes they had "entrancing visions" and "lovely ideas."

In 1800 he wrote, "As nitrous oxide . . . appears capable of destroying physical pain, it may be used to advantage during surgical operations in which no great effusion of blood takes place."

And Michael Faraday, another remarkable young scientist, who was for a time Davy's assistant, experimented with ether as well as laughing gas. In 1818 he wrote, "When the vapour of ether is mixed with common air and inhaled, it produces effects very similar to those occasioned by nitrous oxide."

Here, plainly, were the clues that might have led to the discovery of the magic sleep. No one followed up these clues. Indeed, because gases did not really cure disease and had a bad effect on some patients, doctors stopped using them completely. They were too dangerous, doctors said; only quacks would use them.

The Pneumatic Institute was shut down. Davy and Faraday went on to make important discoveries in chemistry and electricity, and gave up experimenting with gases that could relieve pain.

One English doctor, Henry Hill Hickman, did not give up. He experimented on mice, chickens, and dogs, using carbon monoxide to make them unconscious by suffocation. He was sure the same method could be used on people. Other doctors laughed at him and called him a fool. He kept trying to convince them until in 1830 he died, a disappointed man, at the age of twenty-nine.

And in all the hospitals of the world, patients still shrieked with pain under the surgeon's knife.

3 · Ether and a Country Doctor

Although gases were no longer used by doctors, they were, of course, included in college chemistry courses. Students were delighted to learn that they could become mildly drunk from inhaling laughing gas or ether. Many young people—and some older ones, too—held laughing gas parties and ether frolics. They laughed, they danced, they sang; they hopped and staggered about; they said all sorts of silly things.

Such parties became especially popular in the United States. At the same time, showmen traveled the countryside, entertaining audiences with lectures and demonstrations of laughing gas.

By 1842, ether frolics had reached the village of Jefferson in Georgia. Far from a railroad, surrounded by cotton fields, it seemed cut off from the rest of the world. There were few amusements, and a group of lively young villagers would gather regularly in the home of tall, handsome Dr. Crawford W. Long and sniff ether. And, as a doctor, he began to notice something strange.

Often, after inhaling ether, one of his friends would accidentally bruise himself, but would show no sign of feeling pain. Often, too, after the effect of the ether wore off, he would find bruises on his own body. He could not remember hurting himself or feeling pain.

"Does ether actually relieve pain?" he wondered. "Could it possibly be used in operations?"

One day he saw the chance to find the answer to these questions. A young fellow named James Venable asked him to remove two small tumors from his neck. Long suggested trying ether, and Venable agreed. Holding a handkerchief soaked in ether to his nose, Venable breathed in deeply. In a few minutes he was asleep. Long quickly removed the tumors, and soon Venable sat up, fully awake.

Long was still not certain about the effect of ether. True, it had seemed to relieve the pain of this operation. But would it work with another?

The answer came when an eight-year-old slave boy was brought to his office. He had burned his hand so badly that two fingers had to be amputated. Again Long used ether. When the boy was asleep, Long amputated one finger. Before he could amputate the other, the effect of the ether wore off. He finished the operation with the boy tied down and screaming with pain.

Long performed several more operations with ether, and each time it did away with the pain. But the search for the magic sleep was not yet over.

For one thing, he was not sure that ether would work in a major operation, and he was afraid to try it. For another, he was beginning to lose patients. There was talk that he was doing dangerous experiments, and people were staying away. Besides, he was only a country doctor,

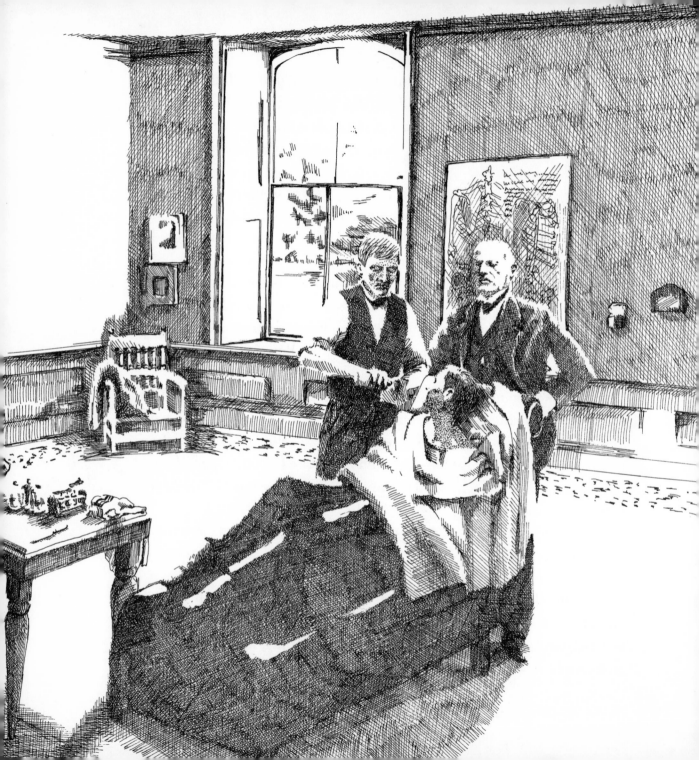

far from hospitals, from universities, from medical libraries. He was not an ambitious man. He had married the prettiest girl in town, he had built up a good practice, and life was pleasant enough. Why change it?

And so he gave up the use of ether, and his patients returned. He made no report to any medical society, he notified no newspaper. He had discovered the magic sleep, but outside Jefferson no one knew; in Jefferson no one cared. It was as if it had not happened at all.

4 · Dentists and Laughing Gas

In 1843, the offices of dentists, like the operating rooms of hospitals, echoed to the cries of patients. Having a tooth pulled, while not so terrible an experience as an operation, was bad enough. Dentists as well as doctors kept hoping for the discovery of a magic sleep.

Two young dentists in Boston, Horace Wells and William Thomas Green Morton, had a special reason for being concerned with pain. They were partners, and they had learned a new and better way to fit false teeth. They had expected that this would bring crowds of patients knocking at their door.

Instead, their patients were few. Their method required that they pull out the roots of all the patient's teeth, and it was simply too painful. Although both men were ambitious and had what Wells called "go-ahead-itiveness," the partnership was a failure.

Of the two, it was Morton who had more "go-ahead-itiveness." A tall man with a bushy, upturned mustache, he had sold books before turning to dentistry and was all business. He had studied at the first college of dentistry established in the United States, and privately with Wells. Now he was determined to make a name for himself and pile up a fortune.

Wells was a gentle, pleasant-faced man with reddish hair and blue eyes. He had taught school, and had thought of becoming a minister, but at nineteen he decided to be a dentist. It was a good choice. He invented several dental instruments and a solder for dental plates, and published *An Essay on Teeth*. He also invented something he called a dustless coal-sifter, and a shower bath for which the water was pumped with the feet. He enjoyed art and music, played the accordion, and collected shells and butterflies.

Discouraged by the lack of patients, Wells dropped out of the partnership with Morton. He left Boston and opened an office in Hartford, Connecticut. There, early in December of 1844, he read a notice in the newspaper:

> A GRAND EXHIBITION of the effects produced by inhaling NITROUS OXIDE, EXHILARATING or LAUGHING GAS! will be given at UNION HALL THIS (Tuesday) EVENING, Dec. 10, 1844. . . . THE EFFECT of the GAS is to make those who inhale it either Laugh, Sing, Dance, Speak or Fight, &c., &c. . . . The entertainment is *scientific* to those who *make* it scientific. . . . Entertainment to commence at 7 o'clock. Tickets 25 cents.

Wells decided to go. He had heard about laughing gas, and he was curious. Besides, it would be amusing, and he could stand a little amusement. And so, on a cold December evening, he and his wife took their seats in Union Hall.

A few minutes later, Gardener Q. Colton—he called himself Professor Colton, though he was only a showman—came out on the stage. He gave a little talk about laughing gas, and called for volunteers to inhale it. A number of men stood up, and among them was Wells.

Mrs. Wells tugged at his sleeve.

"Horace! Please!" she whispered, glaring at him from under her bonnet. She thought it was undignified for a professional man, a dentist, to take part in such an entertainment.

"It's all right, my dear," Wells said quietly.

He strode up to the stage and was the first to take the gas. He inhaled it from a rubber bag with a rubber tube and a wooden spigot. He noticed it had a sweet smell. Almost at once he felt as if he were floating, and he giggled. What he did during the next few minutes he did not know; later his wife told him that he "made a spectacle of himself."

The effect of the gas soon wore off, and Wells sat down on one of the benches that had been placed on the stage. The next man to take the gas was Samuel A. Cooley, a clerk in a drug store. Wells watched him, smiling.

To the delight of the audience, Cooley shouted and waved his arms. He drew himself up angrily, as though he had just been insulted. He punched at the air, fighting an imaginary foe. Chasing his enemy across the stage, he crashed into a bench and cracked his shins. He shouted and waved his arms again. Then, suddenly, he looked around in surprise, and quickly sat down next to Wells.

"Hurt yourself, Sam?" Wells asked.

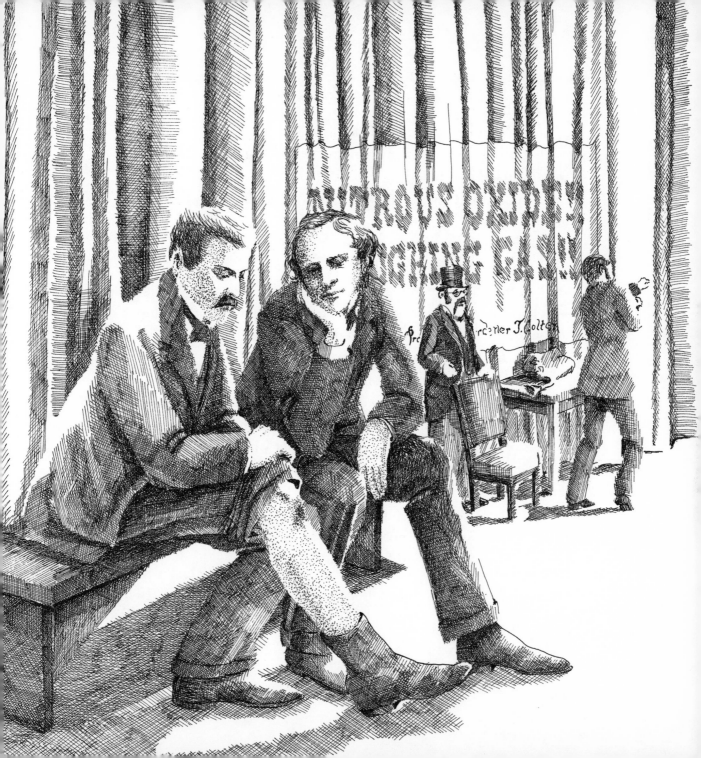

"Hurt myself?" said Cooley. "How?"

"When you ran into that bench," Wells said.

"Didn't feel a thing. But I do now."

He pulled up the legs of his pants and let out a low whistle. His shins were bruised and bleeding.

"Look at that!" he said. "You know, I don't remember running into any bench."

"And you didn't feel any pain? You're sure?" Wells said.

"I told you—didn't feel a thing," Cooley said.

One by one, the other volunteers took the gas. Wells scarcely watched their antics, scarcely heard the laughter and applause of the audience. A single thought repeated itself in his mind: *Sam Cooley felt no pain! He felt no pain!*

As soon as the evening's entertainment was over, Wells hurried over to Colton. He asked if he could have a bag of the gas, and Colton promised to deliver it the next day. After taking his wife home, Wells rushed off to see John M. Riggs, a dentist who was his friend.

Until late that night the two dentists talked. Was it true? Could laughing gas really relieve pain? Only by trying it on a patient could they find out. But how could they do that? It was too great a risk. Too little of the gas might not relieve the pain; too much might kill the patient. How, then, could they find out?

Wells tapped his jaw.

"I will be the patient," he said. "I will take the gas myself, and you, John, will extract one of my wisdom teeth."

The next day both men were in Wells's office when Colton delivered the gas. With him was a relative and Sam Cooley, whose shins had started the whole thing.

Holding the bag of gas, Wells sat down in the chair he used for patients. He opened the wooden spigot and inhaled. In a few minutes the bag slipped from his hands and his head fell back. He seemed to be sleeping peacefully.

Riggs wasted no time. He picked up a forceps, bent over Wells, and began working on the tooth. There was a sharp crack, and the tooth came loose from the jaw. Riggs held the tooth up high so that the others could see it. In a few minutes Wells opened his eyes. He looked as though he was awakening from a refreshing sleep. He spit out a mouthful of blood, then said:

"I felt no more than the prick of a pin."

He and Riggs stared at each other, their eyes wide with excitement. Wells had discovered something new—the magic sleep that allowed teeth to be pulled without pain. Patients would come flocking to them; painless dentistry would make them rich and famous.

As it turned out, things were not quite that simple.

5 · "Humbug!"

Wells learned from Colton how to make nitrous oxide, and he tried it on twelve or so patients. It did not always work, because he did not yet know exactly how much gas to give them. But it worked most of the time, and he felt he could no longer keep his discovery to himself.

Early in January he went to Boston and talked with Morton, his former partner. Morton agreed that Wells should demonstrate his discovery. First, however, they ought to consult Dr. Jackson. A chemist and geologist as well as a physician, Dr. Charles Thomas Jackson was one of the leading scientists in the city. Morton had taken a special course under Jackson at Harvard and was sure he would be willing to advise them.

They called on Jackson in his laboratory. Peering at the two dentists over his spectacles, he frowned.

Wells had given gas by inhalation, had he? Ridiculous! Why, doctors had stopped doing that years ago! It was much too dangerous. Wells was lucky he had not killed anybody. He should forget the whole thing and go home before he made a fool of himself.

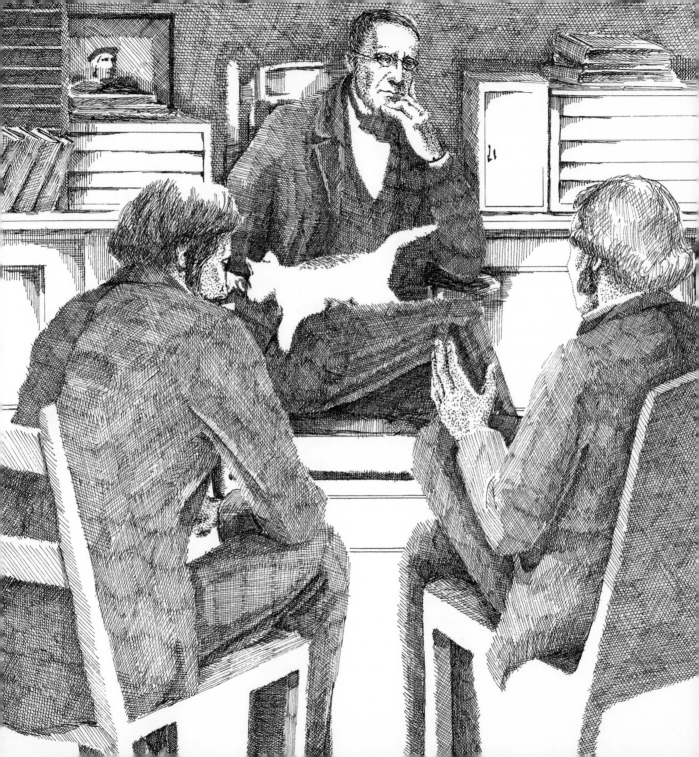

Wells listened politely, but he had no intention of following Jackson's advice. With Morton's help, he arranged to give a demonstration before the medical students and professors of Harvard. It would take place in a classroom at Massachusetts General Hospital, which was the school's teaching hospital. And so, on a gray January morning in 1845, Wells entered the classroom, carrying a bag of laughing gas. At his side was Morton, who was to be his assistant.

Dr. Warren, the chief surgeon of the hospital, introduced Wells to the small crowd of doctors and students. It was easy to see that Warren was not at all hopeful. Too many people had come to him with new ways to relieve pain. Each had proved worthless, and he was sure the same thing would happen today.

Wells made a short speech, explaining how he had used the gas. He then gave the gas to his patient, a student who had volunteered to have a tooth pulled. The patient breathed deeply and lay back in the chair, fast asleep.

A hush came over the room. Using a forceps he had borrowed from Morton, Wells quickly pulled the tooth. As it came loose from the bone, the patient groaned.

One of the doctors laughed.

"Humbug!" yelled the students. "It's a swindle! A fake!"

Shouting, booing, stamping, they forced Wells to leave. The patient awakened and was surprised to find that the tooth was already out. He could not remember groaning.

He tried to tell the others that he had felt no pain, but they would not listen. They had heard him groan, therefore he must have felt pain. Wells's method was a humbug. He was a swindler, a liar, a cheat. Angry and disgusted, they wanted no more of Wells or his laughing gas.

Outside the hospital, Wells said to Morton, "I removed the gas bag too soon."

And when he returned to Hartford, he told a friend, "They wouldn't believe me, but just the same this idea of mine will be used in all great surgical operations inside of five years."

6 · Morton, Jackson, and Ether

The months passed, and few people in Boston remembered Wells and his laughing gas. One of the few was Dr. Morton. Like all dentists, he saw that dentistry could make little progress until a way was found to relieve pain. There was another reason, too, why it was important to him, as he realized one day from the action of a patient.

She was an elderly woman, and she needed a complete set of false teeth. But that meant all her own teeth had to be pulled, and she would not allow it.

"No, no, Dr. Morton," she said. "Impossible. I couldn't stand the pain."

And she walked out of his office.

Morton was anxious to build up a large practice, and he hated to lose a patient. It was fear, of course, that drove people away—fear of pain. If only there was a way to make dentistry painless! Why, the man who discovered it would make a fortune!

If only there was a way. . . . Perhaps there was something in Wells's method, after all. Hadn't it worked in a number of cases? Then why had it failed in Boston? Could it be that Wells was right when he said he had removed the gas bag too soon?

Morton decided it was worth looking into. He would get some laughing gas from Jackson and try it on his own.

True, Jackson had warned Wells against using the gas—but he was in some ways a strange man. Although he was a medical doctor, he had never practiced medicine. He had turned instead to chemistry and geology. He had studied in Europe as well as in the United States, taught at Harvard University, and was widely known as a chemist.

In 1832, returning from a stay in Europe, he met another passenger aboard the ship, Samuel F. B. Morse. Morse was a painter and inventor, and the two men had a number of talks about electricity and magnetism. Shortly after, Morse announced his invention of the telegraph. Jackson immediately claimed that he had given Morse the idea. It took Morse seven years to prove that there was nothing in Jackson's claim.

Morton found Jackson in his laboratory, as usual. Jackson was sorry; he had no laughing gas on hand. And if Morton wanted to experiment with gases, why didn't he try sulphuric ether?

"Ether?" Morton said. "What is it—a gas?"

Jackson told him ether was a liquid that gave off fumes which had an effect much like laughing gas.

"Is it safe?" Morton asked.

"Safe enough," Jackson answered.

He himself had inhaled ether once or twice. It had put him to sleep for a while, and had done him no harm. Morton could get all the ether he needed at Burnett's pharmacy.

During the following weeks, Morton spent most of his time experimenting with ether—or so he later said. He went off to his country house in West Needham, where, he insisted, he used ether on his dog, on goldfish, on beetles, worms, and caterpillars. He also claimed that he experimented on a few people, including himself.

But Morton never offered any proof that he had done these things, and much of what he said seemed too far-fetched to be true. Exactly what he did in those weeks never became clear. There was never any doubt, however, about what happened on the last day of September, 1846.

On that day Morton was in his office with another dentist, Dr. Grenville G. Hayden. They were discussing ether, wondering whether they could risk trying it on a patient. Around six o'clock the door swung open and a man with a swollen jaw walked in. He was Eben Frost, a music teacher. He had a toothache, a terrible toothache, and could wait no longer to get the tooth pulled. But, like most people, he was afraid of the pain.

"Doctor," he said, "can't you give me something for this tooth? How about this mesmerizing I've been reading about?"

"I have something better than that," Morton said.

It had grown dark, and he asked Hayden to bring over the lamp. He seated Frost in the dental chair, took out a handkerchief, and soaked it with ether. He held it under Frost's nose and told him to breathe in deeply.

In less than a minute Frost was asleep. While Hayden held the lamp above him, Morton pulled the tooth. Another minute or two passed. Frost awoke, saw the tooth on the floor where Morton had dropped it, and said that he had felt no pain.

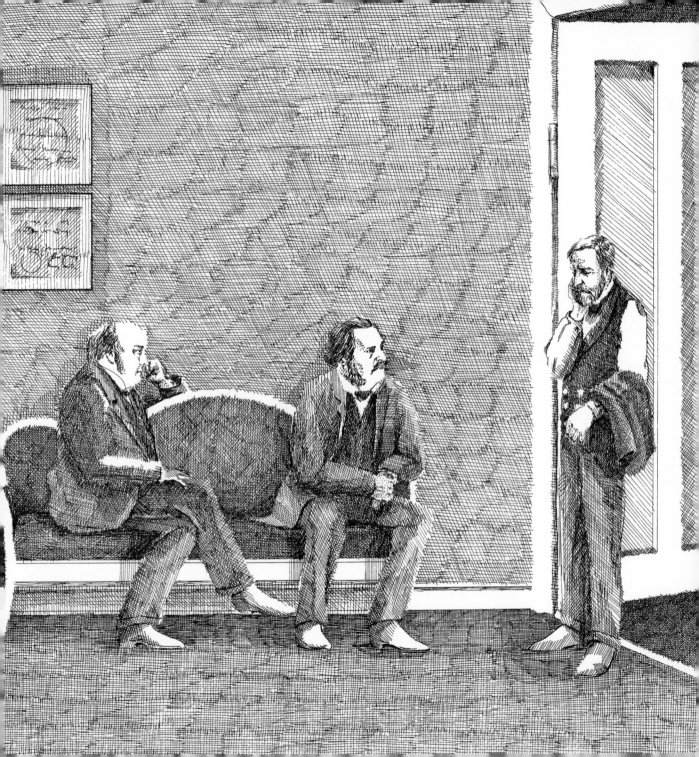

The three men talked excitedly for a while, then Morton had Frost sign a statement of what had happened. Hayden signed it, too, as a witness. That same evening Morton hustled Frost and Hayden to the office of the *Daily Evening Journal*. The next morning the paper carried this story:

> Last evening, as we were informed by a gentleman who witnessed the operation, an ulcerated tooth was extracted from the mouth of an individual without giving him the slightest pain. He was put into a kind of sleep, the effects of which lasted for about three-quarters of a minute, just long enough to extract the tooth.

Morton wasted no time in planning his next step. He would patent his method of relieving pain; anyone who wanted to use it would have to pay him a fee. When Jackson heard of this, he demanded a share of the profits. It was he who had told Morton about ether. Without his advice, Morton would never have made his discovery.

At first Morton refused, but in the end he gave in. He also agreed to put Jackson's name on the patent application. Jackson in turn agreed to assign his rights in the patent to Morton.

It seemed like a friendly arrangement, but it was the beginning of a feud that Jackson would carry on even after Morton's death.

7 · This Is No Humbug

Morton had every reason to be satisfied with himself. He had discovered the magic sleep that made painless dentistry possible. And once he had been granted a patent, the money would roll in. He would be rich as well as famous.

But why stop with dentistry? Why couldn't ether be used in surgical operations? The more he thought about it, the more certain he was that it would work.

Feeling very sure of himself, he called on Dr. Warren at Massachusetts General Hospital. He explained everything about his method except that he had used ether. He intended to keep that a secret until he had been granted a patent. In talking to Warren, he said he had used a mixture, preparation, or compound; in his application for a patent, he called the preparation "Letheon," a word he had invented.

Warren listened closely. Morton's method sounded promising. But so had many others—and they had all failed. There had been so many disappointments, so many humbugs. And a surgical operation was not

35

Hammond Public Library
Hammond, Ind.

the same as pulling a tooth. Suppose Morton's method failed. Suppose the patient died. Could they risk a man's life?

On the other hand, what if this were really the magic sleep doctors had been hoping for? If this method really worked . . .

For a few moments Warren was silent. He rubbed his big nose. From under his bushy eyebrows he looked around the room, as if searching for the answer. Then he spoke. He would take the risk. The next time he operated, he would try Morton's method. He would let Morton know as soon as he scheduled an operation.

While waiting to hear from Warren, Morton went to an instrument maker with a sketch for an inhaler. It would allow him to give the gas more conveniently and to control the flow.

The inhaler was to be a glass globe with two small necks. One neck would be left open to admit air. In the other neck would be a wooden tube with a tap. The globe would be filled with ether, and the patient would put the end of the wooden tube in his mouth. Breathing through his mouth, he would inhale a mixture of air and ether vapor.

Before the inhaler was finished, Morton received a message from Dr. Warren. He was invited to demonstrate his discovery on Friday, October 16, 1846, at ten o'clock.

On the morning of that day, doctors and medical students took their places in the operating theater of the hospital. The patient, Gilbert Abbot, was seated in an operating chair. He was to have a tumor on the right side of his neck removed by Dr. Warren.

A little before ten o'clock, Warren spoke briefly. He said that in this operation he would test a preparation which Dr. Morton, a dentist, claimed would make a patient free from pain. A murmur came from the audience of doctors and students, and then there was silence—deep silence.

Five minutes passed, and Morton did not appear. Warren took his watch out of his pocket and stared down at the seconds ticking away. Ten minutes passed, fifteen—and still there was no Morton. Warren frowned with annoyance and disappointment.

"Since Dr. Morton has not arrived," he said, "I presume he is otherwise engaged."

There was another, louder murmur from the audience, this time punctuated by laughter. Of course! Morton was just another faker, like Wells and the rest. He must have realized that the doctors would see through his little scheme and decided to stay away.

Slipping his watch into his pocket, Warren turned to the patient and picked up a knife. At that moment there was the sound of footsteps at the door. Morton burst in with a package under his arm, followed by Eben Frost. They were both out of breath.

Morton apologized for being late. The instrument maker had not finished the inhaler until the last minute.

"Well, sir, your patient is ready," Warren said.

Carrying the inhaler, Morton went over to Abbot.

"Are you afraid?" he asked.

He pointed to Frost, saying that he had inhaled the preparation and had not felt any pain.

"No," Abbot said. "I feel confident, Doctor, and will do exactly as you tell me."

Morton stood behind Abbot and placed the tube of the inhaler in Abbot's mouth.

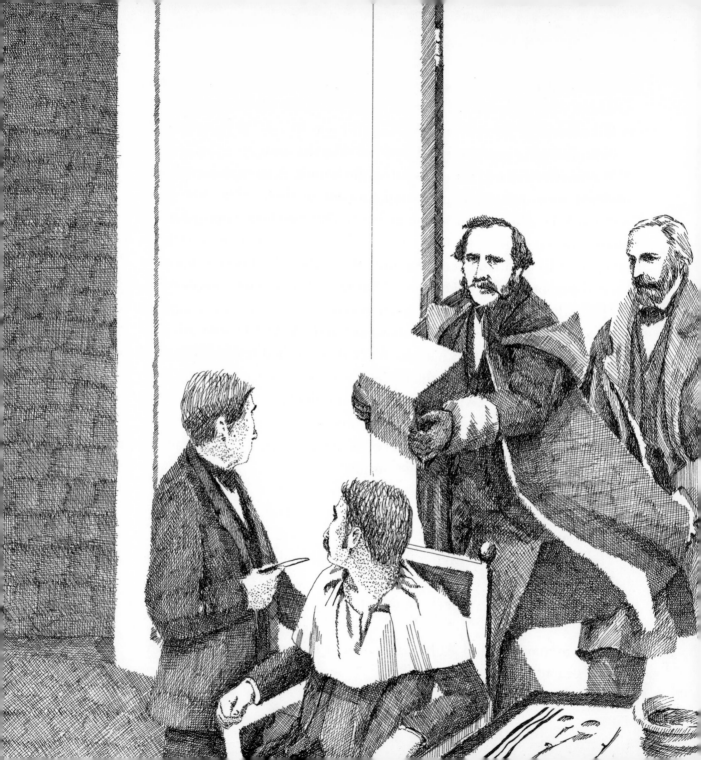

"Take a deep breath," he said. "Breathe in, deeply and regularly."

Abbot's eyes closed. He stirred, muttered a few words, then seemed to fall asleep.

"Dr. Warren, your patient is ready," Morton said.

Warren nodded and began to cut out the tumor. Again the doctors and students were silent. They leaned forward in their seats, watching, waiting. Was this, at last, the magic sleep they had been hoping for? Or would Abbot suddenly shriek and yell like any patient during an operation? But Abbot, too, was silent. When the operation was over, he opened his eyes and looked around, as though in a daze.

"Did you feel any pain?" Warren asked.

"No, it didn't hurt at all," Abbot muttered. At first he had felt as if someone were scraping his neck. After that, he had felt nothing, and had pleasant dreams.

Warren faced the amazed doctors and students.

"Gentlemen," he said, "this is no humbug."

8 · Alice Mohan's Leg

On November 7, 1846, a crowd of doctors and medical students gathered at Massachusetts General Hospital. As they waited for the doors of the operating theater to be thrown open, they talked about Morton's preparation. It had been used in three operations, twice successfully. In the third operation, the patient had felt pain. All three operations were simple—minor operations, the doctors called them.

The operation that was to take place today was different. A young woman named Alice Mohan was to have a leg amputated. This was a major operation, and extremely painful. Would Morton's preparation stand the test? Would it keep Alice Mohan peacefully asleep while the surgeon cut off her leg?

And what was Morton's preparation? It was a fluid, of course, whose vapor was inhaled by the patient. Letheon, Morton called it. And what, exactly, was Letheon?

Morton did not deny that it was mainly ether; but said that he had improved it by adding several things. The truth was that he had only been trying to disguise the ether to keep it a secret. What he added did no more than color the ether and slightly mask the odor. But the crowd of doctors and students did not know this, and one of them said:

"Ridiculous! How can we use the stuff when we don't know what it is? It's against the rules of medicine to keep anything a secret!"

As a matter of fact, the doctors on the staff of the hospital, especially Dr. George Hayward, had felt the same way. They demanded that Morton tell them what was in his preparation, and he finally agreed. He wrote a letter stating that it was ether, but insisted that the letter not be made public. And so, to the crowd that came to witness the operation on Alice Mohan, Letheon remained a mystery.

At last the doors were opened, and the crowd rushed into the operating theater. Every seat was taken, and some of the students had to stand. An hour or so went by, and the crowd grew impatient. The doctors kept pulling out their watches; the students stamped their feet and made loud remarks. Where was Dr. Hayward, who was to perform the operation? Where was Morton? Where was the patient?

They were behind a closed door, in a room just off the operating theater. Alice Mohan lay on a couch. Near her stood Morton, Warren, Hayward, and still another doctor on the staff of the hospital, Henry J. Bigelow. Hayward had refused to use ether unless Morton made a public announcement of what was in his preparation. Morton argued with him, and neither man would give in.

"Gentlemen, we are getting nowhere," Bigelow said, and drew Morton aside.

He talked long and earnestly, until Morton finally said, "All right."

Bigelow then went into the operating theater and read Morton's letter to the audience. A few minutes later, Alice Mohan was wheeled in. After Warren gave a brief talk, explaining why the amputation was

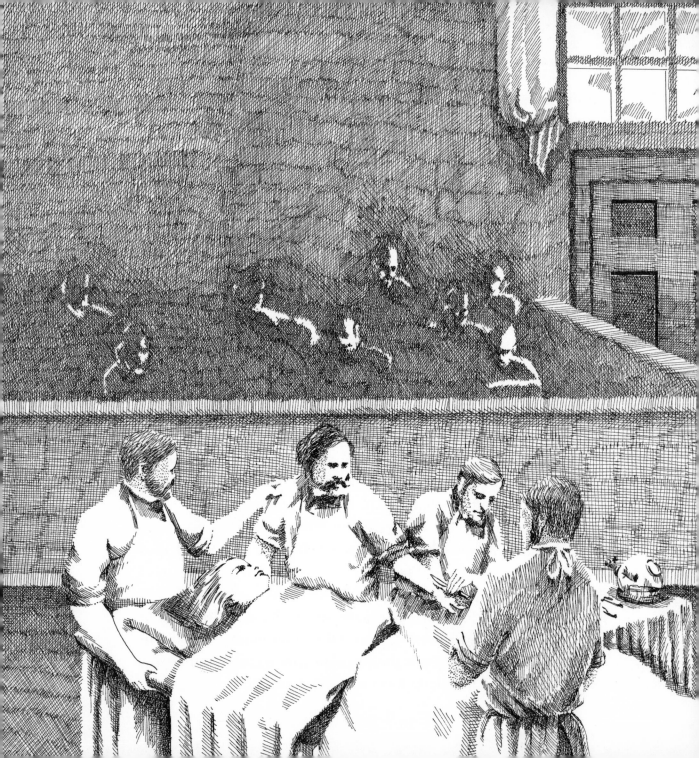

necessary, he called on Morton to give the patient the ether. Soon she was asleep, and Hayward began the operation. When he had amputated her leg, Warren twitched her sleeve.

"Alice!" he said. "Alice!"

Opening her eyes, she said, "Sir?"

"I guess you've been asleep, Alice," Warren said.

"I think I have, sir."

"Well, we've brought you here for an amputation. Are you ready?" Warren asked.

"Yes, sir," Alice answered. "I am ready."

Warren held up her amputated leg so that she could see it.

"It is all done," he said.

A roar of applause rose from the bank of seats and echoed from the high, domed ceiling. Morton's method had passed the test of a major operation.

There could no longer be any doubt about it; here, at last, was the magic sleep that did away with pain during operations. But what should it be called? It needed a name, a scientific name—and Dr. Oliver Wendell Holmes, who was famous both as a physician and as a writer, came up with it.

In a letter to Morton, he suggested that the sleep be called "anaesthesia," with the adjective "anaesthetic." It was based on a Greek work meaning "without feeling," and he spelled it in the Greek manner. Later it was generally spelled "anesthesia."

Holmes urged Morton to settle on the name, because it would be repeated "by the tongue of every civilized race of mankind." Morton took his suggestion. Everywhere the magic sleep was called anesthesia, and whatever caused the sleep was called an anesthetic.

9 · The Blessing and the Curse

"I have seen something that will go around the world!"

These words were spoken by Dr. Bigelow after he witnessed the amputation of Alice Mohan's leg. He soon proved to be right. News of anesthesia quickly spread from Boston to other American cities, and then to Europe. Operations under ether were performed in England, France, Germany, and Russia.

For Morton's discovery meant even more than the relief of pain, important as that was. It meant that surgeons no longer had to rush through operations; they could take their time and go more and more deeply into the body. They could perform complicated operations never before thought possible.

Doctors everywhere realized that anesthesia had opened up new fields of medicine, and from everywhere came praise:

> *This is the most wonderful discovery ever made. . . . A glorious victory for mankind. . . . This is the most important and greatest discovery of our century. . . . This is*

*the greatest blessing, a gift from heaven, one for which we
owe the utmost gratitude to the discoverer. . . .*

There was glory enough for all the men who had played a part in this wonderful discovery. For Morton, who had brought anesthesia to the attention of the world; for Jackson, who had suggested the use of ether; for Wells, who had shown how to use inhalation and laughing gas; for Long, who had actually performed the first operation under ether.

And yet, to each of these men, during their lifetime, the discovery brought more grief than glory. What was a blessing to the world was to them a curse, and the first to feel the full weight of the curse was Horace Wells.

After his failure in Boston, Wells returned to Hartford. He went on experimenting with laughing gas, but he was a sick man. His illness forced him to give up his dental practice, and he turned to other things. Among them was organizing a scientific exhibition in Hartford. In December of 1846 he sailed for Paris. His plan was to buy paintings and engravings, which he would then sell in the United States. Besides, he believed that the long voyage would be good for his health.

His health did improve, and he was able to carry out his plan to buy pictures. But he was amazed to find that all Paris was talking about anesthesia. Jackson had already written to the French Academy of Sciences, claiming to be the discoverer; the French knew of Morton and of Wells, too, from magazine and newspaper articles.

What was even more amazing, Wells was given a hero's welcome. He was the guest of honor at banquets and parties; he spoke before scientific societies. He was the man of the hour—but the hour passed. A friend urged him to send in his claim, like Jackson, to be the discoverer of anesthesia. If the French scientific societies recognized him as the real discoverer, so would the rest of the world. He must go home, gather up his proofs, and make his claim.

Wells took his friend's advice. Back in Hartford, he got statements from witnesses of his use of laughing gas. He made his claim in a short pamphlet with a long title—*A History of the Discovery of the Application of Nitrous Oxide Gas, Ether, and Other Vapors to Surgical Operations*. He was immediately attacked by Jackson and Morton. Of course Wells was not the discoverer of anesthesia! It was impossible because nitrous oxide was not a safe anesthetic!

Wells knew they were wrong. He would show the world that laughing gas was a safe anesthetic. He would show them something else, too. While in France, he had learned about chloroform. Its effect was much like that of ether, and many European surgeons were using it in operations. Wells decided he would introduce chloroform to the United States, where it was then unknown.

Thinking he could do better in another city, Wells left Hartford and went to New York. He rented an apartment on Chambers Street, where he experimented on himself with chloroform. But no matter how he tried, he could interest no one in his ideas on anesthesia. As the weeks went by, he found that only by getting drunk on chloroform could he forget his troubles. One week in January of 1848 he took even more than usual.

Half in a daze, he wandered out into the evening. The gathering darkness and flickering lights made everything unreal, as if he had

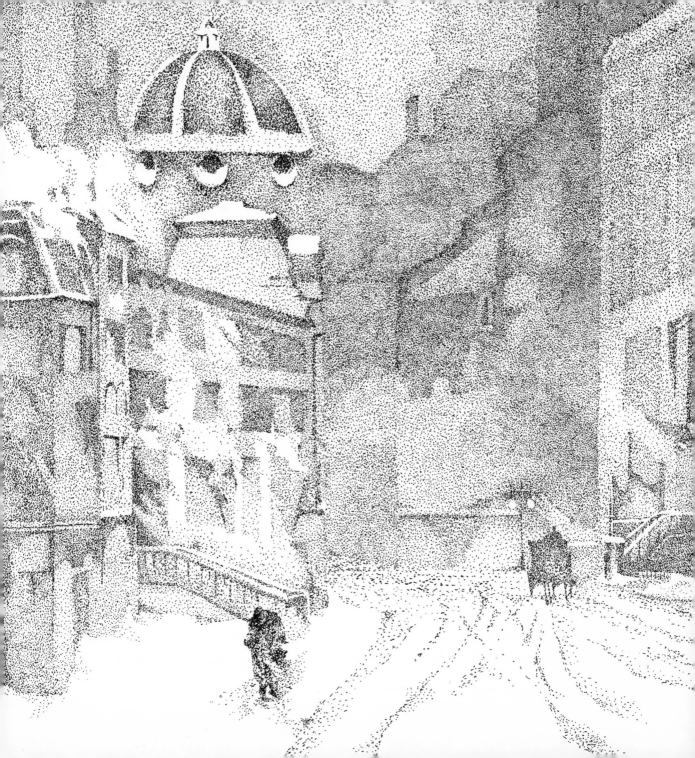

come to a strange, mysterious land. Aimlessly walking the streets, he fell in with one of the men who seemed always to be hanging about Broadway.

This man told Wells his girl had sprinkled acid on him and ruined his clothes. Now he wanted to do the same to her. Wells took him to his apartment, gave him a vial of acid, and the two went looking for the girl. When they saw her on Broadway, the man sprinkled acid on her shawl.

"Hey! This is all right!" he said to Wells. "Let's do it to some others!"

"No," Wells said, and, taking back the vial of acid, went home.

All that week Wells inhaled chloroform. On Friday, in his own words, "I lost all consciousness before I removed the inhaler from my mouth. On coming out of the stupor I was exhilarated beyond measure . . . and seeing the vial of acid standing on the mantel, in my delirium I seized it and rushed into the street and threw it at two females."

Luckily, the women were unhurt; the acid only spotted their clothes. They screamed and caught hold of him, and a policeman came running up. His mind fogged by chloroform, hardly knowing what was going on, Wells was hauled off to prison.

Alone in his cell, he thought, "I must be going mad," and felt that his brain was on fire.

There was only one way to put out the fire. Calling the guard, he asked if he could go to his apartment and pick up a few things he needed. Strangely, he was given permission, and soon returned to his cell. In his pocket was a straight razor and a bottle of chloroform.

Sunday night, by the light of a candle, he wrote two letters. In one, to the public, he confessed his crime. In the other, to his wife in Hartford, he wrote, "I am fast become a deranged man. . . . I cannot live and keep my reason, and on this account God will forgive the deed. I can say no more. Farewell."

Around midnight he sat on his bunk. He poured the chloroform over his handkerchief, and put it over his nose and mouth. To hold it in place, he put on his hat. He picked up the razor, snuffed out the candle, and breathed in deeply. Just as he was losing consciousness, he cut the artery in his left thigh. Quietly, as the blood drained from him, he slipped into sleep and then into death.

A few days later, a letter for him came from France. The Paris Medical Society had voted that to Wells was due the honor of having first discovered and successfully applied the use of gases whereby surgical operations could be performed without pain.

10 · Benefactor of Mankind

Less than two weeks after the operation on Alice Mohan, Morton was granted a patent for his method of anesthesia. Now, he felt, he was well on his way to fame and fortune. He would win his fortune by selling licenses to doctors and hospitals for the use of his inhaler.

It happened, too, that the United States had gone to war with Mexico. Surely the army and navy would want to use anesthetics for the men wounded in battle. He would collect fees from the government, and the money would pile up.

The army and navy did indeed use anesthetics, but, to Morton's surprise, he received not one cent. The government believed a scientific discovery like this belonged to the world; it could not be controlled by one man. There was nothing Morton could do about it. Winning a fortune was going to take longer than he had figured. For the time being, he would have to be satisfied with winning fame.

Again Morton was disappointed. Fame could not be won so easily— and one of the reasons was Jackson.

When Jackson learned that there would be no money coming in from the government, he realized that the patent was worthless. He gave up his claim for a share of the profits; there would be no profits. If the government did not pay, there was no reason for anyone to pay.

Jackson did not care about the money. He was not greedy for cash. Although he was known as a scientist far beyond Boston, he hungered for still more glory, for honor, for fame. He wanted to be known as the discoverer of anesthesia, and he convinced himself that he was.

"If it wasn't for me," he said, "Morton would never have heard of ether. He was only carrying out my ideas."

To get support for his claim, he wrote to scientists in a number of countries. He had also sent in a claim to the French Academy of Sciences. So did Morton, and this gave the Academy a special problem.

The Academy had a prize to award, the Montyon prize of 5,000 francs for a "Benefactor of Mankind." There was no question that the prize for 1847 should go to the discoverer of anesthesia. But who, actually, was the discoverer? Morton? Jackson? Wells? The Academy turned the problem over to a special committee, the Ether Commission. The members quickly ruled out Wells; he had done nothing with ether. That left Morton and Jackson. Which was the "Benefactor of Mankind"?

After three years of study and debate, the Commission decided to divide the prize equally between the two men. Neither was satisfied, but Jackson took the 2,500 francs that was his share. Morton turned down both the money and the Certificate of Award, which carried his name and Jackson's.

This left the Academy with another problem—what to do with the 2,500 francs that remained. Finally, the Commission spent the money

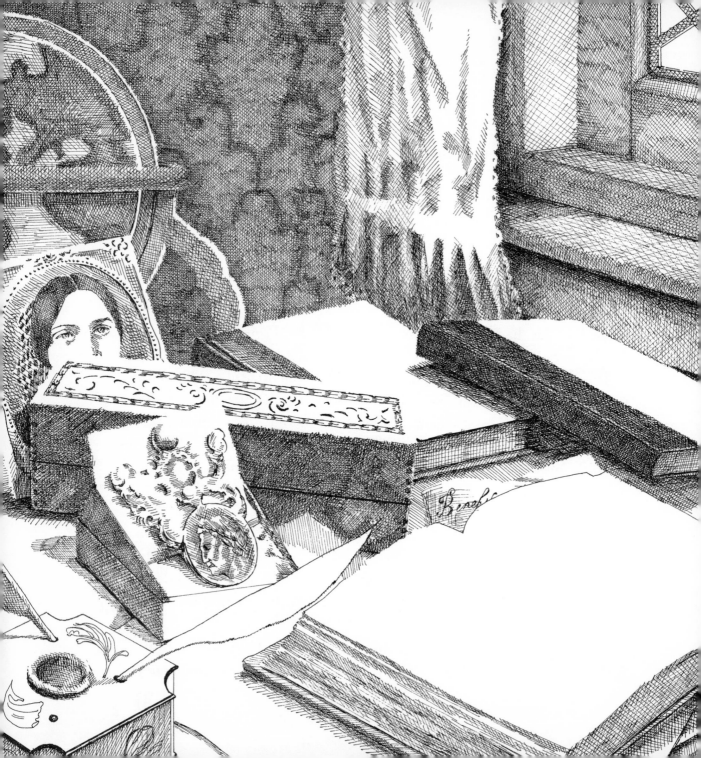

on a gold medal, which was sent to Morton. The Academy had done its duty; it had awarded both "Benefactors of Mankind."

Something similar happened in England. A group of grateful people raised 10,000 pounds to be given to the discoverer of anesthesia. Confused by the supporters of Morton and Jackson, they could reach no decision. They gave back the money they had collected and tried to forget the whole thing.

But even worse was to come for Morton.

He had sold the rights to manufacture and sell his inhaler to a number of businessmen; to a number of others he had sold the rights to collect license fees in certain areas. With his patent worthless, these people demanded their money back. Morton was able to borrow enough to keep them from his door. But his dental practice was ruined, and his health broke down. Closing his office in Boston, he moved with his family to his country house in West Needham.

Morton wrote to Congress in Washington, asking for a grant. He was strongly supported by the staff of the Massachusetts General Hospital. If any man deserved to be rewarded by the government, they said, that man was Morton.

Many congressmen agreed, and a committee recommended that he be given $100,000. But again there was confusion. Jackson loudly insisted that he, and not Morton, was the discoverer. Both men hired lawyers to carry on the fight. Morton spent his summers farming in West Needham; the rest of the time he made many trips to Washington, where he talked to congressmen and government officials. This took money, and believing he would be awarded $100,000, he borrowed heavily. He was soon deeply in debt.

The battle between Jackson and Morton began in 1847 and went beyond Congress. Noted men took sides, signed petitions, wrote letters. It looked as though Morton would win out, when Senator Truman Smith of Connecticut spoke up for Horace Wells. Smith said the honor should go to him and the money to his widow. Then Senator Dawson of Georgia brought up still another name—Dr. Crawford W. Long. A few more doctors also turned up, each claiming that he had been the first to use ether, even before Long.

For fifteen years the congressmen investigated, debated, considered, reconsidered. Jackson saw that he had little chance to gain the reward. To keep it from Morton, he threw his support to Long. Completely bewildered, the Congressmen could reach no decision. They simply gave up and dropped the whole matter.

Meanwhile, trying to protect his patent, Morton had started several lawsuits. In 1862 he was again struck by a crushing disappointment; the Supreme Court ruled that discoveries like his could not be patented.

Meanwhile, the Civil War had begun. Although Long was against the South leaving the Union, he served as a doctor for the Confederate army. Exactly what Morton did during the war never became clear. His son later claimed that Morton gave ether to hundreds of wounded soldiers, but there were no records to show that this was true.

One thing, however, was clear: Morton was a broken man.

11 · Three Deaths

In his house at West Needham, Morton tossed restlessly on his bed. It was no use; he could not sleep. Day or night, he was so nervous he could not lie or sit for long in any position. And the slightest surprise, the slightest noise, could bring on an attack. He would grow weak and dizzy, while pain shot through his body, piercing his arms, his legs, his back, his head.

Sitting up in bed, Morton stared at the window, still black with night. He had given the world the magic sleep of anesthesia—and he could not sleep.

How could he? He was a poor man now, and owed thousands of dollars. Almost every day someone came knocking at his door, demanding money he could not possibly pay.

Nobody seemed to care. Congress had turned against him. Except for a few old friends and the doctors at Massachusetts General, so had everyone else. They were saying that he had done a terrible thing by getting a patent and trying to profit by his discovery. They were even saying he had not really discovered anesthesia.

Nonsense! He, Morton, was the discoverer, the only true discoverer! Long was a fool, Wells had died a madman, and Jackson—

"Jackson!" he cried aloud. That liar, that swindler, that evil, scheming devil who had fought him every inch of the way! And he was still at it!

From the table beside him he snatched up a magazine. It had come by mail from New York the day before, and contained an article claiming that Jackson had discovered anesthesia. With a shout of rage, Morton flung the magazine across the room.

Well, he wasn't through yet! He would fight back! He would show Jackson! He would show them all!

In the first light of dawn he got out of bed and began to dress. He told his wife he was going to New York. He would make the magazine print the truth. Sooner or later, the world would proclaim him the discoverer and give him his just reward.

"But you're not well," Mrs. Morton said. "And there's no need to go. You could write to them and—"

"No," Morton said. "You can't stop me, Elizabeth. No one can stop me. I'm going."

When he arrived in New York the city was in the midst of a heat wave. From the blazing sky the heat poured down, overflowing every street and alleyway, every building, like a flood of fire. Almost at once Morton had a bad attack. A doctor was called in, and a telegram was sent to his wife in West Needham. On the fifteenth of July she was at his bedside with two doctors. They advised getting a trained nurse, and ordered that Morton be bled and ice put on his head.

Morton refused to follow the doctors' orders. As soon as they left, he got out of bed. If only he could escape this heat! It surrounded him, weighed down on him, clung to him and clogged his lungs and nostrils.

"We're going out, Elizabeth," he said.

A relative had lent them a carriage; they would ride to Morningside Heights, where they might get some relief from the heat.

In the fading light of evening Morton drove the carriage up Broadway and turned into Central Park. Even the darkness gathering under the trees brought no hint of coolness. There was no wind. Not a leaf fluttered; the trees might have been made of stone.

Near the north end of the park, Morton suddenly dropped the reins and jumped from the carriage. He began to run toward the lake, as though he were about to plunge into the water.

"William, William! Come back!" Mrs. Morton called.

He came back to the carriage, drove on a short distance, then jumped down again. Running to a fence, he leaped over it and fell to the ground.

"William!" Mrs. Morton called once more.

Morton did not answer. He lay there, silent, not moving. Mrs. Morton hurried to his side, and some people who were passing by clustered around her. One of them ran for help, and soon an ambulance took Morton to St. Luke's Hospital. In less than two hours, on July 15, 1868, he died.

When the news reached Jackson, he was filled with hope.

"Now that that ignoramus will no longer be around to tell his lies," he thought, "everyone will realize that I discovered anesthesia."

To his amazement, nothing of the sort happened. Morton and Wells,

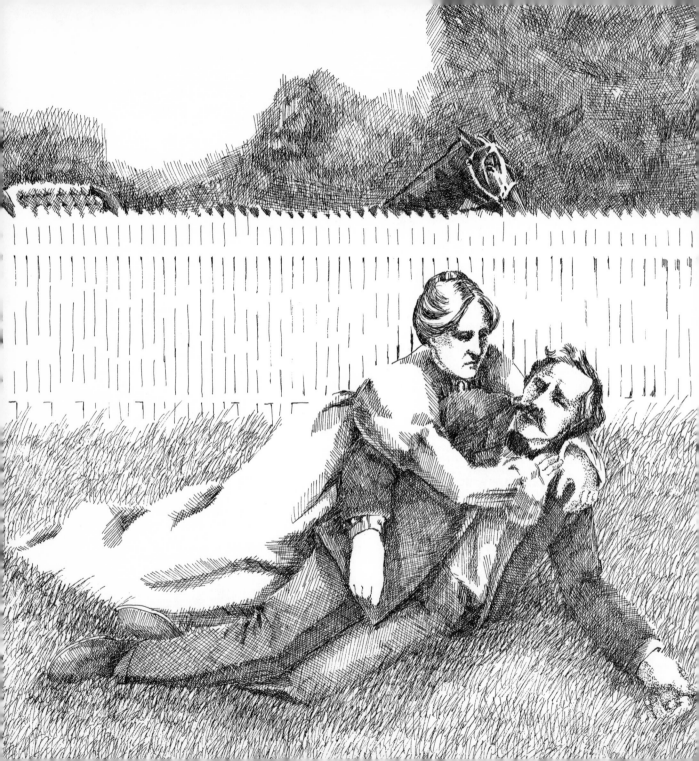

Morton and Wells—those were the names most often linked with anesthesia. Long, too, had his supporters. As time went on, people seemed to forget about Jackson.

He tried to remind them. He wrote letters to scientists and to scientific societies: he sent articles to newspapers and magazines. No one was interested, and Jackson could not understand it. Was he to be pushed aside for two mere dentists, for two stupid pullers of teeth?

No, no, no! He had to prove that he, and he alone, was responsible for anesthesia. Nothing else mattered. They had thrown out his claim about the telegraph, but by God, they weren't going to cheat him of this, too! He could think of nothing else, and slowly, slowly, his other thoughts seemed to be slipping away from him—or, rather, it was his mind that was slowly slipping from him, and one day it gave way altogether.

He was pronounced insane and sent to the McLean Asylum.

While Jackson was spending his days behind locked doors and barred windows, Long was quietly going about his business as a doctor. At the end of the Civil War he returned to Georgia and his medical practice. He had been a country doctor, and a country doctor he remained. Except for the war, he had had a good life. And yet, there was a shadow over his final years. He might have given the world the gift of magic sleep, and he had pushed it aside.

One day in 1878 he was called to the home of a woman about to give birth to a child. Standing at her bedside, he suddenly staggered and fell. He was carried into the next room and laid down on a couch. As the child was born, Long died of a stroke.

Two years later, Jackson died. For the last seven years of his life he had been in the asylum, a lunatic among lunatics.

59

12 · The Honor of Silence

The men who had given the world anesthesia were dead, but the battle over who was the real discoverer went on.

The state of Connecticut, especially the city of Hartford, insisted that it was Wells. Massachusetts, especially the city of Boston, insisted that it was Morton. Georgia, especially the city of Jefferson, insisted that it was Long.

Each of the cities put up statues and monuments to honor its particular hero. The town of Plymouth in Massachusetts even displayed an old rocking chair with this label: *Seated in this chair, Dr. Charles T. Jackson discovered etherization February, 1842.*

Meanwhile, doctors found new anesthetics and combinations of anesthetics. Besides ether, chloroform, and nitrous oxide, they used ethylene and cyclopropane, divinyl ether and cyprome ether, morphine, cocaine, Novocain, pentothal. They learned to make an anesthetic from curare, a poison which the Orinoco Indians of South America daubed on their arrowheads.

They learned other ways of giving anesthetics besides inhalation—by enema, by injection into a vein, by blocking off nerves. They could put patients into a deep sleep or make only one part of the body insensitive to pain with a local anesthetic. There was so much to know about anesthesia that anesthesiology became a medical specialty in itself.

And, while the patient slept, surgeons could perform operations never before possible. They could do open heart surgery; they could remove and replace organs, such as kidneys; they could do things that in the past would have been called miracles.

For years the battle over the discovery went on; books, articles, research papers, speeches were the weapons. Slowly most of the facts fell into place and it became clear what part Morton, Wells, Jackson, and Long had played.

To Morton went most of the credit for the discovery. Although his hope had been to make money, it was he who had brought anesthesia to the attention of the world, and the inscription on his bust in the Smithsonian Institution in Washington honors him as The Discoverer of Surgical Anesthesia.

But the highest honor of all, for Morton and the rest, is silence—the silence in every operating room in the world. No longer are these rooms filled with the terrible screams and cries and groans of suffering patients; no longer does the knife that heals give pain.

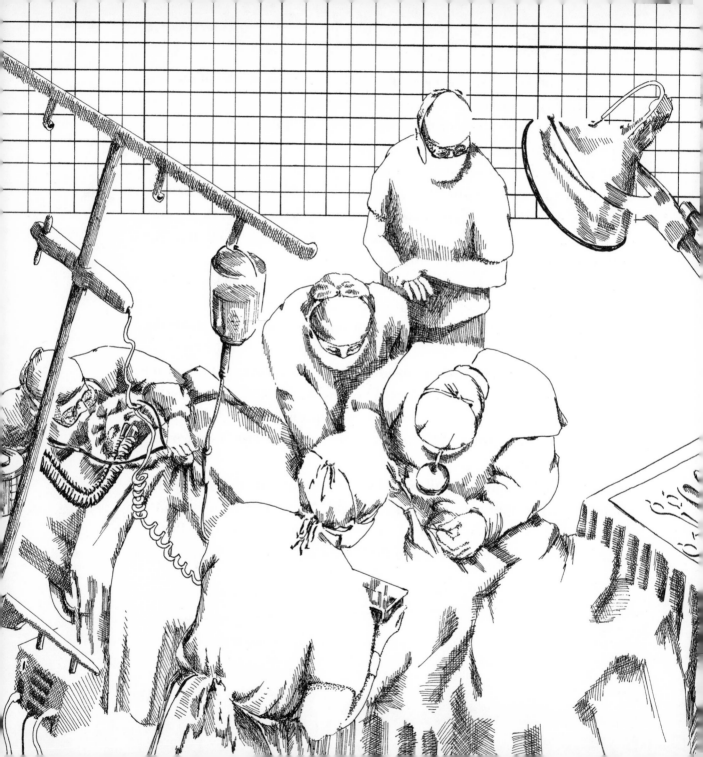

SOME PEOPLE TO KNOW ABOUT

HUMPHREY DAVY (1778-1829)   English scientist who made many notable discoveries in chemistry and physics, and invented the safety lamp for miners.

MICHAEL FARADAY (1791-1867)   English scientist; his discoveries in chemistry and physics, particularly in electricity, are among the most important in the history of science.

OLIVER WENDELL HOLMES (1809-1894)   American physician and writer of poems, essays, and novels.

FREDERICK ANTON MESMER (1733-1815)   German physician who used what he called "animal magnetism" to hypnotize his patients. This method of treatment became known as "mesmerism."

PHILIPPUS AUREOLUS PARCELSUS (1493-1541)   Swiss chemist, alchemist, and physician. Many of his ideas were far in advance of his time.

JOSEPH PRIESTLEY (1733-1804)   English minister and scientist whose experiments laid the basis for modern chemistry.

JOHN COLLINS WARREN (1778-1856)   American physician, one of the founders of the Massachusetts General Hospital and its chief surgeon.

SELECTED BIBLIOGRAPHY

Flexner, James Thomas. *Doctors on Horseback: Pioneers of American Medicine*. New York, The Viking Press, 1937.
    The last sixty pages deal with the discovery of anesthesia, but contain many inaccurate statements.

Fülöp-Miller, René. *Triumph Over Pain*. Translated by Eden and Cedar Paul. Indianapolis, The Bobbs-Merrill Co., 1938.
    This book is generally considered to be biased and untrue to the facts. The author was more concerned with constructing a dramatic story than in setting down what actually happened.

Haggard, Howard W. *Devils, Drugs and Doctors*. New York, Harper, 1929.
    A history of medicine for the layman.

Raper, Howard Riley. *Man Against Pain*. New York, Prentice-Hall, 1945.
    Written in lively fashion, this book includes a study of the controversy about the discovery of anesthesia and a critical bibliography.

Robinson, Victor. *Victory Over Pain*. New York, Schumann, 1946.
    An authoritative book on the search for anesthesia.

Smith, Philip. *Arrows of Mercy*. New York, Doubleday, 1969.
    The story of the development of curare as an anesthetic.

Hammond Public Library
Hammond, Ind.